HOW TO LOSE WEIGHT

Secrets to Weight-loss Revealed

By James Adewola

TABLE OF CONTENTS

Introduction

Losing weight is one of the most popular searches
on the Internet. All over the world, there are literally
thousands of people who are interested in losing weight.
Some want to do it because they want to look better,
while others are more interested in physical fitness
and health. Regardless of the reason, you have to
understand that there is a right way to lose weight.

There is no need to resort to complicated surgeries
or pills that have unwanted side-effects.
In this book, you will discover information that is
going to motivate you to lose weight in a natural and
healthy manner.

From the start, it should be mentioned that losing
weight is very much related to your mindset. If you
put your mind to it, then you can do it. There are
variety of valuable information you will learn in
this book that would help you lose weight, including
music, a change in the diet and physical exercise.

You will learn how you can drink more water and lose
weight, learn cooking tricks that actually promote weight
loss and specific methods on how to burn belly fat on a
daily basis.

Everything that is presented here will teach you that you can lose weight naturally, reducing the health risks that are commonly associated with obesity and increasing the level of your fitness.

In order to get started with losing weight, you need to understand why it is so important you achieve this objective. Apart from the aesthetic reason, which is obvious to everyone, you need to think about the medical conditions that are associated with obesity.

The list is long but it includes cardiovascular conditions, diabetes and bone problems. Hypertension is the number one associated factor with obesity and it can have long term consequences; losing weight through natural methods can help you avoid such problems and stay healthy for a long period of time.

Motivation is highly important for losing weight, as you will have the opportunity to discover below. Once you are motivated, you will find yourself working really hard to achieve your goal.

The important thing is that you do not try to lose a big number of pound all at once; make smaller and realistically achievable goals. In this way, you can enjoy the success of each step that you achieve and be proud of yourself.

Once you achieve a milestone, you will find an even greater strength to continue with your battle against the extra pounds.

Motivation Tips

If you have decided that you want to lose weight but you cannot seem to find your motivation, be sure to read the following tips. You will soon discover that you have the inner strength to lose weight and look amazing.

Once you start on the path of losing weight naturally, you are bound to want to stop at some point. If you reach such a point, be sure to give these motivation tips a re-read and you will be just fine.

Set a big goal – let's say you want to lose 30 pounds and break it down into smaller and easier-to-achieve goals. You might say that this is not helpful but it will actually make your life so much easier.

Choose and write down on a notebook paper three big reasons for which you want to lose weight. Repeat them every time you feel like you are less motivated. They will guide you through the losing weight process.

Start the losing weight program with another person

if possible but not mandatory. For some people, it is easier to go through such a process, if they have someone else going through the same thing. Plus, this person will keep you motivated at all times.

Avoid temptations. If you want to lose weight, then be sure to stay away from temptations of different sorts. Once you eliminate those from your life, you will feel more motivated.

Do not put your trust in over-night losing weight solutions. These are just scams and they often do more harm than good. Stay motivated by choosing to lose weight naturally.

Choose a pair of pants which doesn't fit anymore and keep them at hand for motivation. Do not be too drastic in your choice and keep a realistic track of your progress.

Start your weight loss program at the start of a season, such as spring. The weather is beautiful, the air is warm and everyone is wearing nice clothes.

That for one is sure one good reason for one to be motivation, as we all want to look beautiful and fit as well.

Take photos of your achieved goals. Start by taking a photo at the beginning of the weight loss process and then take several photos to track your progress.

You will see how amazing it feels to have lost even a couple of pounds. Talk about motivation, right?

Mindset

A wise man once said that if you put your mind to something, then you will certainly achieve your goals. Setting your mind to help you lose weight is not an easy task to accomplish, but it is not impossible.

You have to educate yourself in avoiding temptations and also to stop using food as a way to cover up emotions, negative thoughts of piling frustrations.

The mind can be freed so much, once you learn that food should only represent nourishment for the body and nothing more. You are the only one responsible for choosing the right mindset for losing weight.

If you want to lose weight in a natural manner, then you need to set your mind first. Visualize an image of how you will look in the future, after you would have lost the excessive weight.

Organize a mental list with new activities that you will

be starting once you have lost the weight you wanted. Set up a motivating phrase and repeat it on a regular basis.

This can be like your own credo and it can help during the hardest phases of the process, such as the night cravings or passing by a certain temptation.

The interesting thing about the mind is that it can be tricky. As you will proceed with the weight loss process, you will notice that it will becomes increasingly difficult to resist temptations.

Sometimes, the mind can be tricky by suggesting a little bit of temptation and nothing more. Surely, you don't want to fall for the temptations because if you do, you will end up wanting more and more.

However that may not necessarily be the case for you, as you have already gone through a good part of the weight loss process and you are more capable of resisting temptations.

Take a small bite out of a chocolate, eat a small piece of candy or several french fries. You will suddenly feel the power to go on.

The educative process of the mind takes time but it is highly rewarding in the end. Learn how to concentrate on the positive aspects of losing weight, organizing a list of benefits. Make sure that you do not lose sight of these positive aspects, otherwise your mind will immediately focus on the bad and the hard ones.

No one goes through a pleasant process of losing weight but the important thing is that you end up winning the war. Never allow your mind to drift in the wrong direction.

Find things that motivate you and repeat them in your mind on a regular basis. Learn how to correctly handle negative emotions, stress and frustration. Remember, your mind is a valuable tool!

Music and losing weight

Ever since the ancient times, it has been said that music is food for the soul. That could not be truer in a world that is so stressed and filled with negativism.

You might not have thought about music as an ally or strategy that could help you lose weight, but the truth is that it is very effective and can help you a lot.

Avoid sad music that makes you want to eat ice cream and feel sorry about yourself. Choose music that makes you feel alive and prepared to look fantastic again.

Music often sends a message. If you choose the right music, then you will feel motivated to lose weight, without even knowing it.

There are certain songs which are perfectly written for movement and these are the perfect help when you are feeling down.

Music may be food for the soul, but dancing on this music is the best way to lose weight. Plus, you will feel great while dancing and listening to your favorite music. This is the kind of physical exercise that you do out of simple pleasure and you know that for certain.

Everyone says that losing weight is hard and it is actually a painful process. Throughout that process, you can find things that are going to make your life easier and music is one of them.

It will help you get up when you are feeling down and it will remind you why you wanted to lose weight in the first place. At the same time, it will provide you with the energy you need to get moving and dance.

Dancing is one of the best ways to exercise and it provides so much pleasure.

There is a strong connection between music, losing weight and the mind. Studies have shown that humans experience has a powerful release of endorphins when they participate in activities for pleasure. These endorphins are happy hormones and they can contribute to weight loss.

It will reduce internal reactions that triggers negative emotions and stress. Dancing to your favorite music can guarantee an explosion of endorphins; once you dance, you will contribute to your goal of losing weight and feel happy at the same time.

Make sure that you establish a music routine that you can dance to for losing weight. Choose songs that are vibrant, filled with positive tunes and listen to them on a regular basis.

Dance like you mean it and allow yourself to get rid of all the accumulated tension. Soon, you will see the results in your body as well. Music is a helpful ally in the battle against excess weight and you should use it quite often.

Dieting

Everyone knows that, in order to lose weight naturally, a change in the diet is required. However, changing the diet does not mean you should stop eating altogether.

Refraining from eating can generate other health problems and you do not want to have to suffer or deal with that moving forward so It is for the best that you follow a balanced diet. Try focusing your diet supplements with food that is solely based on fresh fruits and vegetables.

Increased consumption of fruits and vegetables will transform and increase the level of your metabolism which in result turns your body into a fat burning machine.

When it comes to dieting, you will see that there are certain things you are allowed to eat and just as many you should stay away from.

Let's start with the things you are not allowed to eat, which you probably know already. The most important thing is that you refrain from eating foods with a high glycemic index.

 Processed foods, sugary drinks and fast food are also on the top list to avoid. Avoid eating excessive quantities of carbohydrates, or you will never lose weight.

Everything that is heavily processed, fatty or excessively refined will add unwanted pounds and it will prevent you from losing weight sooner. Sweets are the worst and they are the biggest temptation.

Now, let's move on to what you are allowed to eat. When it comes to fruits, you need to pay attention to the quantity.

Although they are highly beneficial and nutritional for our consumption, But we have to eat in moderation.

Also, keep in mind that the fruits should be consumed fresh and not added to other sweets. There are certain fruits, such as watermelon, that should be consumed in reduced quantities (high sugar content).

Other fruits, such as pineapple, stimulate the fat burning process, so they are highly recommended. Try to eat fruits which are in season, as these are the best for your health.

As for vegetables, try to consume them fresh and raw. Eat plenty of salads during your weight loss program but make sure that you avoid heavy dressings, as these are empty calories you do not need.

Grilled vegetables are also recommended, as they retain all the flavor and healthy nutrients. Avoid frying vegetables, as they will lose their nutritional value.

Dieting is hard at first but once you set up your diet schedule, things are going to be easier. Try to eat at home and not in a restaurant, where there are plenty of temptations.

Drink plenty of water with your meals, as it will give your stomach the sensation of satiety and it will help you eat less. You can also visit a nutritionist and obtain a diet adapted to your personal needs, or blood group.

Exercising

Losing weight can become a natural process, especially if

include physical exercise on your to-do-list. If you have a long period of absence from exercising, then you should start out slowly to avoid strenuous physical exercise especially in the first few days.

Keep in mind that you will also be on a diet, so your body might feel all these changes as being a bit too much. Start by taking a walk around the block then if you feel up to it, do a little bit of power walking.

The trick with physical exercise is finding the type that is to your liking. A lot of over weight people have forgotten that physical exercise is fun; however, it is never too late to learn once more about the benefits of physical exercise.

There is one very important thing that should be mentioned here; do not expect to lose weight without physical exercise or applying some type of aerobic activity on your schedule.

You need movement to get your blood pumping and make your heart stronger; you need movement to regain your physical and even mental fitness.

Just as with the diet, if you plan on exercising to lose weight, it is important to establish a routine. If you are a morning person, then exercise in the morning and take advantage of the peace and quiet.

Do a set of easy exercises and stretch before going to bed.

If possible take advantage of the decent weather outside to jog, ride a bike or play tennis. Don't think of physical exercise as something imposed; try to find physical activities that make you feel good.

Remember what sports you used to be good at and try them again. If there is a certain sport you have always wanted to try, there is no better time than the present to do that.

You can use the desire to lose weight as the perfect excuse to purchase a new bike, to go skiing or swimming. It is not important what kind of physical exercise you actually choose; what matters is that you will get your body accustomed to movement once more and feel amazing, while losing weight at the same time.

When your body is physically active, your mind is stimulated as well. Physical movement is responsible for the production of happiness hormones, which significantly help with losing weight.

Set your mind to exercise on a regular basis and be sure to follow the same routine, so that you obtain the maximum efficiency from the work out process. Combined with an adapted diet, physical exercise is going speed up the process and tone your shape while you lose weight in a natural and efficient way.

Drinking water

A large percentage of the human body is represented by water. Paradoxically, if you do not drink enough water, your body is going to retain water and add extra pounds. Often times, people take pills that promise a slimming effect and they become frustrated when they notice the pills didn't deliver the expected results.

These pills are bad for health and they eliminate water from the body, leaving it dehydrated. Instead of going through all that trouble, it is for the best that you drink enough water to prevent dehydration.

There are a lot of people who say that they drink water only when they are thirsty. This is one of the biggest mistakes you can make and you need to learn to drink water even when you are not thirsty. It is for the best to establish this helpful routine, just like everything else.

When you wake up in the morning, drink a glass of water and allow your internal organs to be activated. Make sure that you drink at least eight glasses of water every day.

Apart from that, you can also drink tea (unsweetened) and natural fruit juices (in moderate quantities, as they contain high levels of sugar from the fruits).

Water is also important during meals. If you drink a lot of water with your meals, then you will trick your stomach into thinking it is full. Thus, you will eat lesser quantities of food and you will lose weight faster in a natural manner.

You need to make a commitment to yourself to drink water often, even if you don't feel like it. Don't wait until you are thirsty, as this means the body has already reached a high state of dehydration.

Also, avoid replacing water with other liquids, such as coffee, soda pops, sugary drinks or smoothies. Coffee may give you energy but it will dehydrate the body quite a lot, so you might want to avoid it.

When you do your physical exercise routine, make sure that you have a bottle of water around. Don't drink large quantities of water at once but rather take small sips, making sure that you replace the water lost through physical effort.

In addition, at night, you need to make it a habit to drink water. Keep a bottle by your bedside and drink a few sips during the night.

Drinking enough quantities of water is essential for losing weight. If your body is hydrated, then the puffiness sensation is going to be reduced as well and you will feel amazing.

Cooking tricks

If you want to lose weight, then you need to learn how to cook at home. Once you start cooking for yourself, you can choose foods that are healthier and reduced in calories.

Below, you will find several cooking tricks that are going to be quite useful in the kitchen. Make sure you read them carefully and try them in real life.

- Go shopping and purchase all the basic things that are needed in a kitchen. In this way, you will be able to prepare a delicious and healthy meal as soon as you get home (no more ordering in).

- Arrange your cooking tools and learn their purpose. If you have everything you need, then in a short period of time cooking will become a pleasure.

- **Learn the healthy ingredients you should have in the kitchen. The list includes but is not limited to:**

- Fresh fruits and vegetables (frozen are allowed as well, as they can be stored for prolonged periods of time), yogurt, cheese, lean meat, eggs, rice, pasta, whole grains, olive oil and vinegar.

- Introduce herbs to your diet. You will soon discover that herbs are not only a healthy addition to any meal but they add a delicious taste.

18

- Make your sauces or dressing at home. Avoid heavy dressings that are store bought, as these contain a lot of calories and they are also filled with preservatives.

Cook your food as little as possible. Eating fresh and raw veggies is going to allow room for maximum exposure of nutrients and vitamins into your body.

Learn how to make the correct associations. For example, refrain from cooking meat with potatoes, as the combination is not good for your health. Instead, be sure to cook lean meat with green veggies and try the stir fry method, as it is quite simple.

For dessert, consider fresh fruits but only in moderate quantities. You can mix them with yogurt for a more delicious taste. Avoid making cakes and other high-calorie pastries.

Learn how to make meals that are colored. The more wonderful a meal is colored, the more you feel attracted to eat it. Choose different colors of paprika, add leafy greens and you will soon see that it works.

Avoid cooking with high-fat products, as these are bad for your health.

How to lose belly fat

Belly fat is most often associated with cardiovascular disease and this is the reason why you need to lose it in a natural manner. Below, you will find a series of recommendations on how to lose belly fat.

Add more proteins to your diet. For example try cooking beans at least once a week. Proteins are easily digested and they help build muscles, as opposed to carbohydrates, which are responsible for the belly fat.

Avoid processed foods that have artificial sweeteners. You might believe that you are protecting yourself from regular sugar, but you are actually causing more problems.

Artificial sweeteners contribute to the belly fat, being one of the primary causes of obesity. Reduce your carb intake, this might sound redundant but it is important to actually achieve this objective. Your abdomen will look fantastic in a short period of time and you will be able to forget about having belly fat.

Include foods with high-fiber content in your diet. These are highly recommended, as they give your stomach a sensation of satiety.

According to a research channeled in the field of nutrition and diet, just 12 grams of fiber a day will help you lose belly fat.

If you like to eat salads, then avoid heavy dressings and go with a light, vinaigrette dressing. Or, if you want, you can simply add freshly squeezed lemon juice to your salad.

Both of these dressings are acidic and they will help you burn belly fat. Never skip a meal. This is highly important, as the body will first start to break down the muscle tissue for energy.

The belly fat is conserved and you don't stand to gain from skipping meals. Do cardio exercises, as these are great for the abdomen.

Eliminate potatoes from your diet, as these actually help the body stored fat, including on the abdomen.Throw out any sugary drinks you might have in the house. These are the worst, as they contain high contents of sugar and they spike your insulin levels, leading to fatty deposits on the abdomen.

Have breakfast each morning. If you manage to do that, then you will feel less hungry throughout the day and you will help your body to lose the fatty deposits on the abdomen.

Post-pregnancy weight loss

All over the world, there are women who are afraid to have children, as they do not want to end up overweight. The subject of post-pregnancy weight loss represents a matter of interest for a lot of women, as they all want to return to

their pre-pregnancy figure as soon as they possibly can. However, the weight loss process should not be rushed and there are several things that can be done in order to promote weight loss in a healthy manner.

We hear so much talk about breastfeeding and how important it is for the baby. Nevertheless, breastfeeding has a lot of benefits to offer the mother as well, for one it will help her lose the post-pregnancy weight to some degree.

Studies performed on mothers of different ages and cultural backgrounds have shown that breastfeeding accelerates the fat burning process. Apart from that, it helps mothers avoid post-partum depression, which can lead to unhealthy eating habits.

If you did not consider breastfeeding as part of your weight loss routine, there is no better time than the present to use it to your benefit.

When choosing the foods for your post-pregnancy weight loss program, consider that what you eat is going to be transmitted through your breast milk to the baby.

This will help you make healthy choices when it comes to the types of foods that you eat. Choose plenty of fresh fruits and vegetables and make sure that you avoid foods that have been overly processed or have high sugar content.

Not only will they make your baby fussy and agitated but they will add on pounds you do not need.

Physical exercise is an important part of the weight loss routine, as regular movement can help you fight postpartum depression and also lose the extra weight much faster.

You can either decide to exercise at home, while your baby is sleeping or the two of you can visit one of those mother and baby centers. In such a center, you will find specialized physical therapists who can help you lose the extra weight and your baby to develop in a healthy manner.

The most important thing is that you do not run out of patience and stay committed to your goals. Losing weight after your pregnancy should not be rushed, especially since your body goes through a recovery period.

Eat healthy, breastfeed and exercise. Soon, you will return to your pre-baby weight.

Men and losing weight

When it comes to losing weight, men need to take a different approach from women. First of all, they have a different metabolism and their necessary caloric intake is higher. These differences have to be taken into account by any by any man who is trying to lose weight, especially if he wants the best results.

Below, you will find a few helpful tips on how to lose weight when you are part of the male population.

Don't follow the same weight loss plan as your girlfriend. Remember, you have different caloric requirements and the weight loss plan she has chosen might not provide the same benefits to you.

Analyze your current physical status in a realistic manner. If you have a good level of fitness but you've put on a few extra pounds, you can go for an intensive physical training program. On the other hand, if you haven't been to the gym in years, it might be a good idea to start out slowly. Maybe walk or perform a light jog for as little as 15 minuted a day.

One of the hardest things to regain is your cardiovascular fitness. In order to be able to lose weight, you need to get your blood pumping again. Sprinting can also be a suitable activity for cardio workouts and it can be done at any moment of the day.

Apart from a strict diet, you need to pick up a sport that offers pleasure. You can lose weight much faster if you start to play basketball or racquetball with your friends. Plus, competition is a known factor to stimulate your desire to lose even more weight.

Learn how to handle stress in a more efficient manner. While women are experts at such matters, men prefer to cover stress and resist the pressure until they can no longer hold out.

Let go off all stereotypes and do something to relieve stress. One of the best examples that can be offered is learning yoga.

The idea is that you learn how to handle stress in other manners than eating out of the fridge at night.

Take photos in order to keep track of your progress. Instead of going up on the scale and checking out your weight obsessively, it might be a better idea to take photos and see the differences.

Train with a friend. This is especially useful when you are having a bad day, as your friend can pick up your moral. Also, a friendly competition doesn't hurt anyone.

Natural home remedies for losing weight

Natural home remedies can represent a helpful addition to your weight loss program, so do not hesitate to try them out. Below, you will find a few suggestions on the best remedies you can use at home for losing weight.

Cinnamon tea
Helps maintain normal blood sugar levels
Recommended 1-2 times/day

Green tea
Fat burning properties
Also contains healthy antioxidants (protection against cancer)
Recommended 1-2 times/day (better on an empty stomach)

Water with rose petals
Recommended because of its diuretic properties

- Keeps the body hydrated

Water with ginseng root and lemon
- Speeds up the metabolism
- Energy boost
- Keeps the body hydrated

Flax seeds
- High fiber content
- Reduce bad cholesterol levels
- Lower blood sugar levels

Honey with ginger
- Recommended remedy for a 'lazy' metabolism
- Fat burning properties
- Keeps the blood sugar levels stable

The best juice recipes for losing weight

Fruit and vegetables juices are your greatest allies against the extra weight. Below, you will find several juice recipes that are simply delicious. Try them out and allow them to work their magic. You can even blend these ingredients at home if you have a blender or juice maker.

#1 Delicious green juice
Ingredients: apples, celery, cucumber, ginger root, kale and lemon

Benefits: contains healthy nutrients and vitamins, stimulates metabolism, and lowers bad cholesterol levels.

#2 Colorful and healthy juice
Ingredients: beet root, cabbage, carrots, lemon, orange, pineapple, spinach

Benefits: detoxification properties, helps the liver metabolize all the extra fat, energy booster.

#3 Healthy juice for a healthy heart
Ingredients: apples, beet root, carrots, lemons and oranges

Benefits: keeps the heart healthy, cleansing properties, high fiber content.

#4 The vitamin cocktail
Ingredients: apples, celery, cucumber, kale, lemons, oranges and parsley

Benefits: high vitamin and fiber content, energy booster, stimulates digestion.

#5 A 'different' lemonade
Ingredients: apples, cucumber, kale, lemons and spinach

Benefits: high vitamin C content, fat burning properties, high fiber content.

#6 A cocktail of roots
Ingredients: carrots, beet root and sweet potatoes

Benefits: cleansing properties, stimulates the liver function, lowers cholesterol.

How to establish a weight loss plan

Wanting to lose weight without having a plan first is like going to battle without any strategy. If you want to come out successful in the end, you need to have a plan and one that works out in your best interest. Below, you will find a series of helpful suggestions that will help you establish your plan.

- Take a calendar and split your weight loss program into weeks. Consider the long term goal and then break it down into smaller, weekly goals.

- For each day of the week, organize your meals. Go shopping and make sure you have everything you need to cook those meals.

- Fill your pantry with healthy snacks and purchase fresh fruits. Use colorful stickers to add the snacks to the calendar. Purchase a membership to a gym that is closely located to your home. In this way, you will not have the excuse that it is too far away.

- Talk to a friend or a group of friends about organizing weekly games at the basketball court (this is just one example; feel free to choose any sport you might like).

- Add a day of the week on the calendar in which you are allowed to eat something not included in the weight loss diet. Use a computer program to track down your progress.

- There are specialized applications that you can also use on your smart phone; you can record the starting weight and track your progress quite easily.

- Organize a list with physical activities (besides the gym) that you find to be enjoyable. Add at least one physical activity to each day of the calendar and make sure that you spend at least half an hour doing it.

- Think about the quantity of water that you need to drink on a daily basis and add stickers to the calendar. Reward yourself with a big yellow start at the end of the day.

- When you have reached the middle of the weight loss program, review your goals. Be realistic about how far or close you are from the big goal and change the remaining goals if necessary.

- Set up a big reward at the end of the weight loss program. It must be something that you really want, so that you really work for it.

29

Organize the weight loss plan so that it is efficient, without being extremely harsh.

General tips on how to lose weight

Throughout this entire book, you have been given specific advice on how to lose weight. This chapter is going to provide general tips on how to lose weight; these can be useful throughout the entire weight loss process and you can always return to them whenever you feel like something is missing.

· Read the label of every product. The rule goes like this: if a product contains more than three ingredients that you do not know, then it is definitely not healthy.

· Watch movies that can inspire you to lose weight. When you will see your favorite heroes doing all sort of physical effort, you will want to try out a few movements yourself.

· For every meal, choose a smaller plate. The smaller the plate, the lesser amount of foods you will be able to digest.

· Avoid prolonged sitting. Try to be physically active as much as you possibly can. Couch potatoes do not lose weight, but they rather add even more pounds to the existing number.

· Choose healthy snacks to keep you lasting between the meals. Crunchy vegetables, pickles, yogurt and fresh fruits etc.

These can kinds of foods all represent healthy snacks you

can consider.

When you get into a restaurant and you are waiting for your order, be sure to ask for a small salad first. This will help you avoid the free bread and other appetizers with high calorie content.

Eat nuts, although they may contain high amount of caloric content however they also offer good calories and fiber that your body needs for digestion and building increasing the level of your metabolism, provided that you do have to be careful of the quantities that you eat.

Apart from that, the consumption of nuts provides an amazing sensation of satiety. Keep a calorie journal. Add every meal and the foods that you ate.

When you see how much calories have added within one single meal, you will certainly want to cut back.

Avoid going shopping when you are hungry. If you do that, your brain will tell you to simply buy everything and you might end up purchasing a lot of foods that are bad for you.

While out shopping, be sure to avoid XXL-sized products and those which are offered at 2+1 offers. These will make you buy more and thus eat more.

If you love a particular snack which is not healthy, such as potato chips, then be sure to buy the smallest bag you can find. In this way, you can have one or two chips, without feeling guilty.

Avoid night-time munching. Sure, you may have gotten accustomed to snacking at night but this doesn't mean you cannot change. Take the light out of the fridge and it will be easier to resist temptations.

Choose a day of the week when you cheat with one thing on your diet. This will make you feel great and it will also keep you focused on your diet. It is far better to cheat this way, than all the time.

Sleep as much as you need. Don't watch television or use your smart phone before going to sleep. You will keep your brain actively wired and you will have trouble going to sleep.

Remember: there is a powerful connection between being sleep deprived and overweight.

Educate yourself to eat more slowly. Often times when we are hungry, we tend to eat quite fast. Drink water with the meals and chew the food really well before swallowing.

This will allow for the satiety sensation to appear faster. Brush your teeth more often, as the minty flavor is often

going to stop you from munching on unhealthy snacks. Also, be sure to floss, so as to maintain excellent dental hygiene.

You might not believe it, but these are all part of the strategies
 that will actually prevent you from becoming overweight.
Watch your weight with increased attention. Step up on
the scale on a daily basis and jot down your values.

This will help you to keep track of your progress and to
have more realistic expectations.

Don't be influenced by others. If someone tells you that
your weight loss program isn't working, don't listen
to that person. The only one that matter is you.

If you are noticing progress, regardless of how small it
might be, then you are on the right track. Always choose
a weight loss program that appeals to you.

Find at least three positive aspects of the program, so that
you are absolutely certain you will not be making all this
effort in vain.

Do not expect results over night. Losing weight takes
time, especially if you want to do it right and make sure that
you stay healthy throughout the process. Give your body
time to return to its fit shape.

33

Conclusion

Losing weight is a battle. If you know how to pick out the right weapons and use them, then you will have no problem winning.

Throughout the process, you might be tempted to give up and return to your old habits. The motivation tips should help you to stay on the right track. Music and dancing are going to help you move from the couch to a standing and active position.

The right diet is going to represent the biggest change you will go through, followed by the physical exercise which is going to fill you with endorphins.

The weight loss process is going to be a period of education, in which you will learn to drink water, to cook healthy and what you should do to lose belly fat.

If you are still not convinced on why you should want to lose weight, be sure to read the following facts on being overweight:

Excess body weight, in combination with poor nutrition and physical inactivity, is responsible for 1 in 3 cancer deaths 6 in 10 adults are overweight or obese.

Only 3 in 10 adults eat the recommended quantities of fruits and vegetables every day.

Medical complications of obesity include: pulmonary disease, liver disease, gall bladder disease, gynecologic abnormalities, osteoarthritis, gout, intracranial hypertension, stroke, cataract, coronary heart disease, pancreatitis, cancer, Diabetes, and venous stasis etc.

Children are just affected by obesity as adults. Studies performed in 2010 revealed that 1/3 of the world's children were overweight or suffered obesity.

1 in 3 kids will eat fast food, 33% of the children watch more than 3 hours of TV every day and only 1 in 3 children have daily physical activities

Because of the staggering increased consumerism, snack portions have increased in size, leading to a higher calorie intake with one serving.

Fast food portions have grown in size, being present at more affordable prices 50% of overweight children are going to become overweight adults.

If you are having a hard time losing weight, then you need to seek out for support and if you have read this book up to this point then you have already acquired a valuable and effective tool in your possession.

Another supporting element you can compliment to combat this process if you need to is the weight loss program on my website http://www.adewolasfitnessconsultants.com.

Use this book as your faithful companion and do not hesitate to apply the advice that was provided here.

Never allow your weight to define who you are; this is a problem you have to handle and it should not become something that leads to excessive anxiety, psychological stress or negative emotions.

Always keep yourself motivated and find ways to be optimistic about your progress; enjoy the small objectives you have manage to achieve and schedule a calendar of all your success.

Never allow someone else to tell you what you can do or how you should look like. The desire to lose weight should come from within and it should be based on your needs to be healthy.

Once you find your inner motivation, you will see that everything else will follow through. Most people don't realize that they make over 200 health-related decisions every day that dictate how well and how long they live.

Every pound that you will lose, will be a sign of victory. And when you will fit into your old pants once more, you will know that you have achieved the big goal.

Losing weight is a process of transformation and you can

come out in the end exactly as the person you wanted to be. Nevertheless, remember that beauty comes from within and it should not only be defined by the physical **appearance.**